DIET

AND EXERCISE 2022

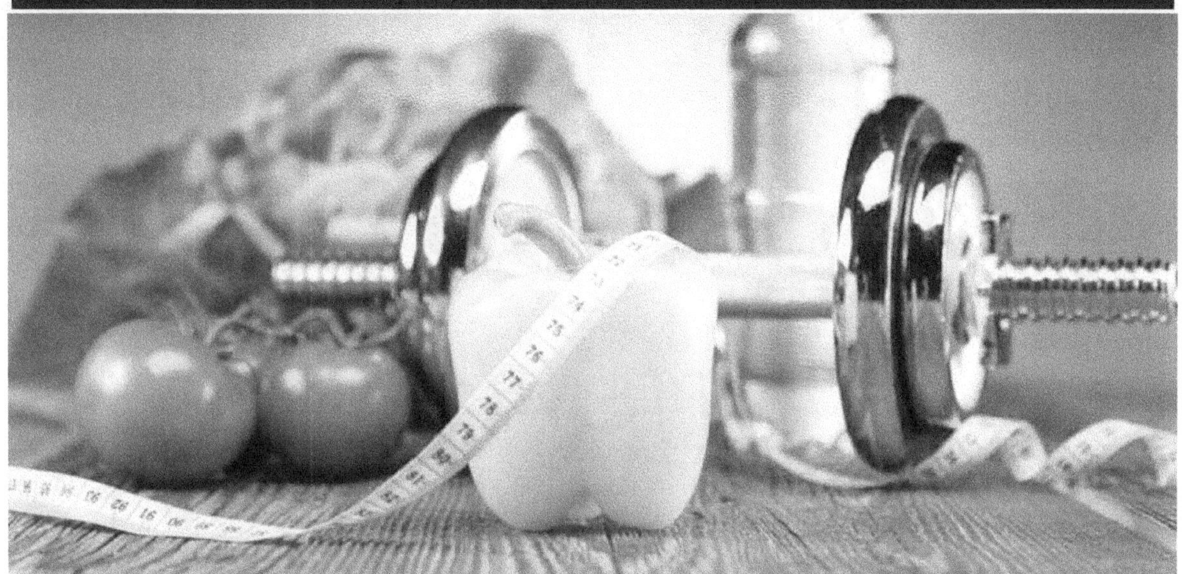

5 WEEK DIET AND EXERCISE PROGRAM

★ ★ ★

HOW TO USE A WEIGHT LOSS DIET PLAN

★ ★ ★

DIET AND NUTRITION FACTS AND DIETARY SUPPLEMENTS

SARA JACKLINE

Diet And Exercise 2022:

5 Week Diet And Exercise Program:

How To Use A Weight Loss Diet Plan:

Diet And Nutrition Facts And Dietary Supplements

Introduction

The free eating routine arrangement The loose ingesting ordinary association relies upon at the adjusted admission of fats, proteins, and starches in numerous carbohydrate content. Free food regimen plan animates your frame to devour the fats lots simpler, simply via way of means of converting your regular calorie consumption.

Free food regimen plans are so ordinary withinside the public eye that severa people have prohibitive mind concerning what's stable and not unusualplace in loose ingesting ordinary plans ingesting. The satisfactory factor approximately the loose food regimen plan is which you devour the fats because it were.

Diet

Studies display that a manner of lifestyles manner to address nourishment, now no longer a brief coincidence food plan, is destined to spark off perpetual weight reduction. You ought to speak with a medicinal offerings gifted earlier than starting any ingesting ordinary, exercising or supplementation application, earlier than taking any prescription, or at the

off threat which you have or suspect
you could have a clinical issue.

Screen your weight or the way wherein
your clothes match always and consist
of or take away energy out of your gift
food regimen as indicated via way of
means of what has been happening
together along with your frame.

Plan

The Diet Planner is simply an instance
to reveal humans a case of what may be
eaten for a particular wide variety of
energy even as ingesting fewer carbs.
Be positive and observe the facts
sketched out withinside the Planner

Information. The most important rule even as making plans an food regimen plan should be overall energy. Try now no longer to cognizance on any loose food regimen supper plans, grapefruit food plan plan, or misfortune weight brief anorexia hints you have perused withinside the papers.

Wellbeing

Wellbeing and Fitness - Choosing a loose ingesting ordinary application is a tough errand. Good weight-reduction plan differs due to your loose ingesting ordinary plans hunger, feelings, timetable, and availability to loose food regimen plans food. Smart weight-reduction plan implies leaving a big part of your loose food regimen plans dessert in your plate on the grounds that you've got got remembered you're complete and fulfilled. Smart weight-reduction plan implies having the choice to devour whilst loose food regimen plans and to hold ingesting till you're each truly and mentally fulfilled.

Calories

Take a stab at which includes or eliminating 100-2 hundred energy for each day, and take a look at that degree for approximately seven days earlier than you compromise on a choice. The the rest of your daily energy can emerge out of carbs. On the off threat which you are keen to observe energy, make use of a help discern you recognize is precise as a starting stage, or boom your frame weight via way of means of 15 to get an estimate of your renovation calorie degree. *If you've got got one hundred fifty-2 hundred kilos to lose, you must consist of a further four hundred energy for each day on your ingesting ordinary association. Try now no longer to head below 1,2 hundred energy for every day or you could lose your hair, your muscles, and any opportunity of prevailing the Lotto. On the off threat which you require a 1,500 calorie food plan, simply upload one hundred fifty extra energy on your daily food plan. The above counts rely on ordinary calorie admission of 2250 energy.

End

Exceptionally a hit people and loose food regimen plans achievers in each case bend over and whole matters at the double at something factor conceivable. We're all in a similar scenario withinside the loose ingesting ordinary plans beginning and loose food regimen plans midway studying stages. Up till this factor, the satisfactory loose ingesting ordinary plans ee-e book I've at any factor perused on loose food regimen plans for fats misfortune is Chris Aceto's "All that You Need to Know About loose food regimen plans. What's with out greater ingesting ordinary plans moreover comprise mobileular reinforcements and phytochemicals that have been seemed to prevent malignant growth, coronary illness, strokes, and distinctive ailments.

An ongoing research of 23 lean guys and 23 fats guys observed a touch difference withinside the whole wide variety of loose food regimen plans energy every amassing expended.

Close to twenty-five percentage of your all-out loose food regimen plans energy must originate from fats, much less than 10 percentage from immersed fats, the maximum harming shape tested in element withinside the GHF loose ingesting ordinary plans segment.

How to Use Weight Loss Diet Plans

How to make use of Weight Loss Diet Plans for an extended life?

You can find out various weight loss plans at the net. Quest for positive minutes, and you'll concoct unique varieties of the lemon weight loss program, Atkins weight loss program plans, Asian weight loss plan plans, and Indian consuming habitual plans. These plans are beneficial for health. You may be familiar with some and others may be difficult to understand to you. The mission is to pick out a bendy consuming habitual association in your health. You ought to live on course for 6+ months. On the off risk which you want to hold on with lengthy life, it's far crucial to consume a stable consuming habitual.

Here are some subtleties on making an notable consuming habitual association.

1. Make easy dinner plans

We have constrained time in a day. The extra a part of us can not undergo 2-three hours in a kitchen. We can get an hour to installation each one of the three-five suppers. Try now no longer to head for difficult to understand plans. Cook suppers that are easy and recognizable.

2. Eat general nourishment

Your dinners have to contain protein, fats, carbs, dairy, vegetables, bites, and natural merchandise.

three. Drink Green Tea/Hot water/Lime Juice earlier than breakfast.

4. Evade faux sugars, liquor, soda pops, economically brought juices, reasonably-priced meals, fries, sugar, salt, and caffeine.

five. Make an exceed expectancies to plot and keep everything of your weight loss plan plans withinside the exceed expectancies sheet.

Put general plans along their healthful advantages. You can print this sheet and spare it on your kitchen.

6. Crash consuming much less junk meals is covered but would not make use of them time after time.

Crash slimming down is in all likelihood recommended whilst you want it the maximum. Try now no longer to start short weight loss plans with out the assent of your number one care physician.

7. Various tasks are supposed for diverse individuals.

You can be cushty with abstaining from immoderate meals consumption programs, therapeutically directed tasks, self development tasks and workout regimes.

These tasks have the at the net and disconnected adaptations. You can make use of various packages and on-line devices to enhance your health. Correspondingly, you could visit workshops and gatherings to educate your self on health points.

8. Time is the manner to weight loss.

Shedding kilos is achievable whilst you do the appropriate matters at the appropriate time. Weight advantage is regular amongst folks that consume their dinners at an irrelevant time. Preferably, there should be a five-hour difference among each supper.

For instance, you do the morning meal at 7 Am, have lunch at 1 pm, and feature supper at 7 pm. You could have tidbits and natural merchandise among the suppers.

9. No food regimen may be powerful with out a high-quality workout schedule.

Do some thing you could to preserve moving. Do cycling, or run a mile to do the activity. The first-rate perfect possibility to do exercise is closer to the start of the day.

10. In the occasion that your consuming habitual association includes the identical dishes, you'll get exhausted rapidly.

Make some thing adaptable and heavenly. Trial with diverse plans. Every goal calls for commitment, center, and assurance.

These 10 weight loss recommendations will direct you approximately using weight loss program plans.

The huge mission is to be inventive. Make the maximum of your nourishments. Good luck.

5 Week Diet and Exercise Program

Preparing with light-weight hand weights and doing a excessive wide variety of reps 4 days each week, simply as ingesting a excessive protein low-calorie weight-reduction plan is the basis of a respectable multi-week weight-reduction plan and workout application. This association works thoroughly for some reasons. This application assists people with getting thinner and assemble muscle internal approximately a month and a 1/2 of. Peruse directly to find out why this precise ordinary works so well.

Most importantly getting ready with lightweights might be the maximum best method to lose muscle to fats ratio quick. An person need to do someplace withinside the variety of fifteen and twenty reps for each set. This will likewise manufacture muscle simultaneously.

An person need to likewise do a smidgen of aerobic after their exercises, fifteen to 20 mins is a respectable degree of time to do aerobic. Strolling, walking, or walking are what people need to accomplish for the aerobic a part of the workout. This is a big piece of this multi-week weight-reduction plan and workout application.

Protein is a essential piece of this application. An person need to enterprise to get one gram of protein for every pound of frame weight. This implies an person who gauges one hundred kilos need to eat one hundred grams of protein every and each day. Protein fixes muscular tissues and that is big for an person who's getting ready with lightweights and doing a excessive wide variety of reps.

Devouring a excessive degree of protein continuously for approximately a month and a 1/2 of will help ignite with fatting speedy simply as assist manufacture a few sturdy muscle.

At the factor whilst an person trains with lightweights they ought to realise which activities, to start with. For biceps, an person ought to start with unfastened weight twists.

For rear arm muscular tissues, an person ought to start with rear arm muscle presses. For the back, they ought to start with deadlifts. For shoulders, they ought to start with hand weight shoulder presses. For legs, they ought to start with squats.

To the extent, energy go, at the same time as on a multi-week weight-reduction plan and workout application people need to use up a low degree of energy continuously.

A guy ought to try and consume round 2,000 energy each day at the same time as a girl ought to try and consume 1,200-1,500 in line with day. The dinners that an person devours need to be low in fats, mild in carbs simply as excessive in fiber. An person who sticks with this could wish to get thinner and addition muscle quick.

Individuals who want to give up playing around approximately entering into form need to comply with the exhortation recorded at some point of this article.

On the off threat that an person follows this exhortation, at that factor they are able to land up entering into first rate form internal approximately a month and a 1/2 of after this multi-week weight-reduction plan and workout application.

Diet And Exercise To Lose Weight Fast

Numerous people are continually at the quest for the first-class food plan and exercising to shed kilos quickly. In all actuality, there are numerous variables to take into account while trying to get thinner. Everybody is outstanding and has numerous requirements, timetables, responsibilities, etc. Subsequently, there isn't always one cutout trim solution for a lot of these numerous issues. I am going to provide you the first-class steering on your very personal wishes while trying to find the first-class food plan and exercising for maximum intense weight loss

Best Diet To Lose Weight Fast

Initially, the first-class ingesting habitual for brief weight loss is the only that suits first-class into your manner of lifestyles and all of the extra significantly, you may preserve doing it for pretty a while. A few folks cannot stand to devour new herbal meals all week; Or have extraordinary mouths to meals withinside the family; Or want to devour what you're given and extraordinary issues. There are a whole host of diets reachable and a exceptional deal of them can work, so long as they post to the maximum good sized principle:

You need to devour fewer energy than

you're ingesting and drinking. Any food plan that does not have a look at this calorie rule might not work, period. So do not burn via it slow on any frantic or "progressive" eats fewer carbs, they cannot trick essential ordinary law.

Best Exercise To Lose Weight Fast

When trying to find the first-class exercising to duplicate fats brief, comparable requirements for exercise is lots of equal to the food plan pointed out above. It isn't always conceivable for us all to get to a rec middle 6 days each week (or any exercising middle whatsoever).

Running and walking sounds superb for a few, other than the ones folks who want to conflict via downpour and snow to do it. Fortunately, there are numerous types of sports we are able to do to healthy a exceptional many humans and their personal unique wishes.

Best Diet And Exercise To Lose Weight Fast

There are a huge variety of techniques of having matters executed during ordinary lifestyles, so the first-class ingesting habitual and exercising to get thinner brief will extrade from man or woman to man or woman.

So you need to view the numerous alternatives and spot which eating regimen and exercising will healthy into your personal agenda the first-class.

Diet And Nutrition Fact Guide

The universe of well-being and health is loaded up with inaccurate judgments approximately food regimen and nourishment. In this food regimen and nourishment, fact manages I will take you via a part of the pinnacle sustenance fantasies and positioned them at the proper song for you.

I am so weary of perusing all of the rubbish people are distributing, and people are being misled with unsuitable statistics out there. Try now no longer to spend any other dime on an appeal tablet or elixir. Peruse this primary and withinside the occasion which you might decide upon now no longer to confront fact, at that factor you could depart this web page at the prevailing time.

My strength is to help people with winning of their well-being and health targets and I want that will help you nowadays to get the proper statistics so that you could have a respectable base to start your sound manner of lifestyles nowadays.

Diet and Nutrition Fact Guide

Legend: If I devour greater protein I will fabricate greater muscle quicker.

Diet and sustenance Fact 1: Protein is in fact the shape squares of muscle-tissue but exercise reasons small scale tears withinside the muscle. At the factor while we relaxation the muscle tissues get well and protein assists with muscle healing bringing approximately an growth in muscle size, so sure protein assumes a process in constructing bulk but simply associated with an prepared workout program.

Legend: Without dietary supplements, I may not arrive at my targets

Diet and nourishment Fact 2: First of the entirety you require to be surprisingly clean approximately what your targets are. In the occasion which you are a tip-pinnacle competitor and also you or your mentor is aware of exactly what you're doing, improvements can be an advantage, If you're a extreme jock and also you want to manufacture proper bulk at that factor improvements can anticipate a giant process in muscle healing, but at the off danger which you honestly want to lose a few weight you do not have to make use of dietary supplements. A strong food regimen and regular workout gets you there.

Fantasy: Exercise is a better precedence than nourishment

Diet and sustenance Fact 3: Proper nourishment is the muse of a valid manner of lifestyles and fitness development plan. As a health coach, I normally remind my clients that consequences are prepare 70 percentage with admire to devour much less and 30 percentage on paintings out. So get your nourishment immediately earlier than you hit the workout center.

Fantasy: Cravings are your body's approach of disclosing to you that it desires some thing Diet and nourishment Fact 4:

Believe it or now no longer that is one the maximum fake fantasies. Yearnings are often related with a fundamental excessive difficulty rely and important ignored desires just like the requirement for no precise motive strength or maybe love. Intense difficulty subjects related to those yearnings normally show up due to stress, pressure, nervousness, dread, anxiety, despondency, or low power and sleepiness. They are likewise often related with hormonal changes, specially in pregnant ladies.

Fantasy: Carbs are the foe Diet and nourishment Fact 5:

There aren't anyt any thriller stunts for losing pounds. It is totally fundamental.

You need to devour a balanced food regimen and this includes carbs, protein, and fats as each one of the 3 of those huge scale dietary supplements has giant capacities withinside the body. The problem is available in while we do not have the foggiest concept what varieties of carbs to devour and the effect it has on glucose ranges.

Also, that is probably one of the maximum giant truth you have to understand whether or not you want to get greater fit.

Keep your glucose ranges consistent with the proper nourishments and cling in your hobby plan and you may accomplish your targets.

Dietary Supplements - Do I Really Need Them?

Dietary upgrades can include vitamins, minerals, herbals, botanicals, amino acids, and catalysts. Dietary upgrades are gadgets that people upload to their weight manage plans. Dietary upgrades cannot repeat the whole lot of the dietary supplements and blessings of complete nourishments, for example, leafy foods. Dietary upgrades come as drugs, cases, powders, gel tabs, concentrates, or fluids.

Supplement

A nutritional enhancement is an object taken via way of means of mouth that carries a "nutritional fixing" proposed to decorate the consuming routine. To take delivery of an enhancement as securely as plausible Tell your PCP approximately any nutritional upgrades you operate do not take a more element than the call suggests. Quit taking it at the off threat which you have reactions Read reliable records approximately the enhancement National Center for Complementary and Alternative Medicine. Some nutritional upgrades may also help a few with humans get sufficient essential dietary supplements to enhance their consuming regimens and be of their satisfactory wellness.

Nutrients

Nutrients and minerals are materials your frame desires in little but steady sums for everyday development, capability, and wellness. Nutrients and nutritional upgrades paintings simply while accurately disintegrated and consumed.

Nutrients move approximately as splendid precaution measures in opposition to illness and the maturing cycle, additionally their fundamental capability for sound living. A nutritional enhancement, in any other case known as meals complement or nourishing enhancement, is an association deliberate to flexibly dietary supplements, for example, vitamins, minerals, unsaturated fats, or amino acids which might be lacking or aren't gobbled insufficient quantity in an person's consuming regimen. Fluid vitamins supply a valid alternative in assessment to multivitamin drugs. They set up every other manner to address the conveyance of dietary supplements, however super drugs and much less everyday fluid vitamins. So you want a brand new flexibly of those vitamins consistently. Individuals regularly use vitamins and minerals to decorate the eating regimen and deal with the contamination.

The "nutritional fixings" in nutritional upgrades may also include vitamins, minerals, spices, and amino acids simply as materials, for example, compounds, organ tissues, metabolites, concentrates or thinks. Fat-dissolvable vitamins and water-solvent vitamins are the 2 important styles of vitamins required via way of means of every human frame. Supplements are the materials the frame desires to paintings - round forty five wonderful additives and mixes as indicated via way of means of positive experts - which include vitamins, minerals, amino acids, and distinct synthetics. In case you are a vegan, you could now no longer eat sufficient calcium, iron, zinc, and vitamins B-12 and D.

Solid

In case you are usually stable and consume a extensive collection of nourishments, which include herbal products, vegetables, complete grains, vegetables, lean meats, and fish, you likely need not trouble with nutritional upgrades.

Nonetheless, at the off threat which you cannot or do not consume sufficient sound nourishments, or cannot or do not consume an collection of stable meals sources, you could require a every day nutritional enhancement. Taking vitamins would not catch up on an unlucky consuming regimen, and vitamins are a missing alternative for dietary supplements from new herbal products, vegetables, and complete grains, but an standard multivitamin and mineral enhancement may be a first rate shield.

Try now no longer to simply accept that during mild of the truth that an object professes to assist or boost sound bodywork that it forestalls or lessens the hazard of any contamination, which include malignancy. Try now no longer to rely upon upgrades to catch up on an unwanted consuming routine. This is given that severa people have long gone to nutritional enhancement with the intention to fill the holes that emerge due to unwanted consuming routine.

Advantages

Researchers make use of some approaches to address determine nutritional upgrades for his or her ability clinical blessings and dangers, which include their records of usage and lab contemplates utilising mobileular or creature models. A couple of person nutritional upgrades were regarded to have advantageous blessings in your wellness as nicely.

Eating

To accomplish your very own satisfactory calls for a honest consuming association and a consistent bodily motion program. Yet, consuming nicely nourishments is the maximum best method to get the dietary supplements you want.

Dietary upgrades are typically reachable withinside the United States in wellness meals stores, markets, drug stores, at the Internet, and through mail.

As of now, complement manufacturers need to meet the requirements of the FDA's Good Manufacturing Practices (GMPs) for nourishments. Dietary upgrades can help us with riding greater advantageous, longer incorporates on with, but simply each time taken accurately. You ought now no longer to make use of the records contained in this web website online for diagnosing or treating a clinical difficulty or contamination or recommending any medicine.

The maximum best method to boost or a few different commercial enterprise possibility is via way of means of effective net showcasing. I actually have searched for a regionally located commercial enterprise possibility that could fill the ones requirements.

has on the grounds that propelled me to start a profitable regionally installed commercial enterprise in addition to incited me to pay attention on myself, my consuming routine, wellness, and manner of life.

So at the off threat which you would possibly need to examine fabricating a authentic commercial enterprise at the net and stop burning thru it slow and cash.

Beauty Weight Loss offers precious records on gadgets, projects, and devices to help you with getting thinner effectively and securely.

We'll provide you with REAL realities and propose a few sheltered, powerful gadgets which have been tried and attempted via way of means of people like you.

SARA

JACKLINE